Following an exercise program does carry a certain level of risk to your health. Before starting this or any exercise program you should consult your physician. You choose to follow the program in this book of your own free will. The author and publisher of this book have no responsibility for any damages you might experiance, personal or professional, as a result of your choice to follow the program in this book.

Introduction

This manual deals with plateau breaking, shock training, and intensity elevation. In this manual I offer the best shock training techniques I have come across. I am sure there are others that I have missed, and many more you can create by combining two or more techniques from the manual. That's great. That's the real point here. Sock training is just that. Shocking the muscle. Doing something differently. Catching the muscle off guard. But remember it just takes the subtlest of changes to get new growth. Less rest time between sets, more reps, more sets, or switching back to a basic 3 sets of 8 to 12 rep routine after a pre-exhaustion, superset, or compound set.

The point I'm trying to make is these techniques are very powerful. A little goes a long way. Most people have the tendency to abuse them and consequently over train. What this means is you erode progress instead of facilitating it. These techniques increase intensity. That means you need to decrease frequency and increase recovery. If you have been doing 3 sets of bench press with 2 minutes of rest between sets, and you decide you want to shock your chest with a pre-exhaustion set of flys followed by benches. Then one or at most two sets is all you will need. Because you are used to 3 straight sets does not mean you are ready for 3 shock sets.

So proceed cautiously. Make little changes and milk them for all they can deliver before going the the next level. Don't specialize on more then one area at a time, and go back to a basic routine after a 4 to 6 week specialization. Remember the specialization routines are meant to allow you to return to your basic routines stronger. After a specialization you should be stronger in the area you specialized on. That means handling more reps and more weight. Do not loose sight of the importance of basic routines and moving heavy weight in basic straight sets. Sock training is meant to supplement your basic training not the other way around. Being able to handle 135 Lbs. for 3 sets of 8-12 reps in the standing barbell curl will yield much greater results then all the super duper arm specialization shock training you can do with 80 to 100 lbs. If you aren't adding weight to the basic compound movements for basic straight sets then you are not progressing.

Shock training while a very powerful tool in your body building/strength training arsenal can be easily abused. Remember once you throw the switch the light is on. Continuing to push on the switch will only break it. If one set is all you needed to trigger growth then 2 or 3 sets won't cause any more and could decrease or stop it. Shock training should shorten and decrease workout duration and frequency. Remember you are trying to do the same or more work as a conventional straight set workout in less time then the conventional workout.

Drop Sets

The Drop Set is simply performing a set of some exercise with your usual heaviest weight for your usual reps, reducing the weight by some amount and performing another set with little to no rest between sets. Generally people do 3 sets in one sequence, but you can do more. And less could be better. There are a lot of variables to play with so let's take a closer look at what can be manipulated.

Number of sets in the break down sequence

2 or more. It's your choice, but think about this. Like I said once you throw the switch there's no point continuing to push on it. So if you are used to 3 sets of an exercise done in straight set fashion with a 1 to 3 minute break between sets then one break down set of 3 or 2 break down sets of 2 would be enough. Don't think because you are used to 3 straight sets that you can do 3 break down sets. Stop and do the math. You just jumped from 3 sets to 9 sets with much higher intensity. A break down set of 100 Lbs. for 12 reps, 80 Lbs. for 10 reps, and 60 Lbs. for 8 reps will make a much greater inroad into your muscle recovery capabilities then 3 sets of 12 reps with 100 Lbs., 80 Lbs., and 60 Lbs. with 2 minutes rest between sets. That one break down set did more for you then the straight sets even though you did less reps in the last 2 sets. Why? Because you were working at a higher fatigue level. At the point that your body is used to you stoping and resting for 2 minutes you go into another set.

Amount of weight decrease between sets

Obviously the more weight you drop the more reps you can get on the next set, and conversely the less weight you drop the less reps you'll get. That's your choice. It depends on your goals. This gives you the chance to have the best of both worlds. For example let's say you are more interested in building size and strength then stamina and endurance. So you start with a weight that allows 5 reps and you only decrease the weight enough that your reps stay between 4 and 6 for you subsequent drop sets. While each set of 4 to 6 reps emphasizes strength and size because you chained together 2 or more sets you are getting 12 to 18 high quality stamina and endurance stimulating reps also.

Amount of reps pre set

Here your goal is to manipulate the weight to get a specific number of reps. This is fine as long as your mind set is to get as many reps as possible with each set and not stop at the targeted number of reps if you can get more. Remember this is shock training. Your goal for these short cycles is to go all out. To take your muscles to a new level. The tendency could be to stop once you hit your targeted number of reps even if you could get more. In my opinion focusing on getting as many reps as possible with each set is a better tactic then having a set number or reps. But have a targeted number of reps in the back of your mind so you have something to shoot for, and have an indicator of when to increase the weight.

Another aspect of this variable is the manipulation of the rep range can be a real time saver. You can hit all the muscle fiber stimulating rep ranges in one break down set and be done. For example your first set can be totally warm-up 25 to 50 reps. The next set 8 to 12 reps. Then a hard 4 to 6 rep. And finish with a 12 to 15 rep flush set.

How to apply to body weight exercises
One of the easiest ways to utilize drop sets with body weight exercises is to go from a harder exercise to an easier one. While this is not exactly a pure drop set. The goal is achieved.

Examples:
Push-ups (feet elevated)->Push-ups (regular)->Modified push-up
Body press->Dip->Push-up
Body press->Push-up->Modified push-up
One leg squat->Two leg squat
Pull-ups->Body rows

With equipment:
Push-ups w/ weight vest/back pack->Push-ups
Pull-ups w/ weight vest/back pack->Pull-ups->Body Row
Use a series of cables. Start with your high resistance and work your way down with less and less resistance. This can be done with most body weight exercises.

Super Sets

A super set is 2 exercises done back to back with out a break. The exercises can be for the same area or different areas. Usually this is done with antagonistic muscle groups. Like bi's and tri's, back and chest, quad's and ham's etc... You are doing 2 exercises per cycle so 2 or at most 3 cycles is all you will need. This is another great way to shorten your workout time.

Examples:
Curls->Tricep extensions
Leg curls->Leg extensions
Barbell row->Bench Press
Press->Upright rows

Bodyweight applications:
Pull-up->Push-up
Hindu squat->Bridge
Sit-ups->Prone hypers
Reverse grip pull-up->Diamond push-up

Giant Sets

Giant sets are chaining 3 or more exercises together that target the same area. One to three times through a sequence depending on how many exercises are in the sequence is all you will need.

Examples:
Preacher curl->Hammer curl->-Wrist rotating curl->Barbell curl
Tricep push-downs->Lying tricep extensions->Close grip bench->Seated tricep extensions
Barbell rows->Pull overs->Pull-downs->Low cable rows
Stiff leg dead lifts->Leg extensions->Leg curls->Squats
Incline bench->Fly->Bench->Pull overs

Bodyweight applications:
Diamond push->Regular push-up->wide push-up
Pull-up->Body Row->Full bridge
Lung->Bootleg squat->Squat->Half bridge

Flushing Set (Giant Set)

This is a specialized version of the giant set. Everything is the same as the regular giant set with one change.   You do 20 to 30 reps per exercise. So you will use 30 to 50% of your 8-12 rep poundages. One cycle would be more then enough. This is a great fallow up to a series of heavy 4 to 6 rep sets.

Bodyweight application:
Obviously with bodyweight you would chose exercises that you can do the high reps with.

Pre-Fatigue

The Pre-fatigue technique doing a single joint exercise and a multi joint exercise that is in the muscle group that the multi-joint exercise works back to back. Two to three rounds is all you will need.

Examples:
Leg extensions->Squats
Pullover->Pull down
Flys->Bench

Bodyweight applications:
Fly hold->Push-ups
Superman hold->Pull-up
Inverted leg extensions->Squats
Bodyweight tricep extensions->push-ups

21's

Do the first half of the chosen exercise for 7 reps, then do the second half for 7 reps, and finish with 7 full range reps. 7 reps is the convention, but you can do this with any rep range you want. 1 to 3 sets is all that's needed. This can be done with any number, and you can change the order of rep segment.

Example:
This can be done with any movement. Weighted or body weight. It is a great way to up the intensity of bodyweight exercises.

11/2 Reps

This is similar to 21's, but done in a different order. For example let us look at how you would apply this to the squat. From the start position go down half way, come back up, go down all the way, come up half way, back down, and return to the top. 1 to 3 set will do the job.

Example:
This is similar to 21's and can be used on any exercise. Like 21's it also is a great way to up the intensity of bodyweight exercises.

Burns

Burns are continuing to do partial reps after you can no longer do full reps. As long as you can move the bar, or in the case of bodyweight exercises do a partial rep, you keep going. You can add a finishing touch at the end by doing a isometric hold.

Example:
This technique is pretty straight foreword. You just keep going until you can not move, and then do the optional isometric hold for a 10 to 30 second. Do not let your form or poster deteriorate to get more reps.

As an example keep doing push-ups until you can just get a couple inches off the floor then push with everything you have without breaking form.

10 x 6

This is a pretty straight forward routine. You are doing 10 sets of 4 to 6 reps. You have 2 choices.   To include your warm-ups sets as part of the 10 or not.   I think including the warm-up sets is the better choice. Shoot for 5 or 6 worksets. You get 1 minute of rest between sets. You push as hard as you can. Do not stop at 6 if you can do more on work sets. If you get 7 or more reps on a set you add a bit of weight. If you get 4 or less reps you take a bit of weight off. The goal is to hit 5 or 6 reps per set, but it is better to truly fail at 4 reps then stop at 6 when you could have gotten 8.

Example:
This is pretty straight foreword for barbell exercises. For body weight stuff you will use the hardest exercises for you, or add resistance to the body with weight vest, bands, or a back pack.

10 x 10

The rules are the same with this routine as the 10 sets of 6 routine. One minute of rest between sets. Go all out on each set. Try to hit 10 reps on each set. If you hit something more add a bit of weight. If you hit less drop a bit of weight. Because the rep target is higher 10 reps I think it is ok to use the first 2 to 3 sets as warm-up and not do extra sets out side the 10. But that is your call. A variation that I want to mention here is combining this tactic with antagonistic super set tactic. For example you might combine low pulley rows with bench press. You will alternate back and fourth between the 2 exercises. You can rest or not, but no more then 1 minute. The point of this workout is to flush the area being worked with blood. I prefer the no rest option. This would mean you should be able to finish 20 sets in the same or less time as it took to do 10 sets with a rest. Remember intensity is all about more quality work in the same or less time. The emphasis is on quality. Be honest with yourself. Leave your ego at the door. You will not be able to handle the same amount of weight with high intensity techniques as you can with straight sets. Other variations of this program are: 10 x 20, 20 x 10, and 20 x 20.

Example:
While the barbell application is pretty straight forward the body weight exercises are the challenge. So we will have to modify a bit. I think 10 sets of 10 reps for pull-ups would be a challenge for most. 10 sets of 10 reps in push-ups is probably not. So try for 10 sets of 15 or 20 etc... Or do 10 sets of max reps, but do not do less then 10 reps per set. Start with harder exercises and change to easier exercises as you are unable to get the 10 reps with the harder one. As far as squats go you should be able to do 1000 straight reps. So if you can not then building up to 10 set of 100 rep body weight squat sets is a great way to get there. If it was me I would not take the 1 minute rest between sets of squats. Instead I would do a circuit of squats, pull-ups, and push-ups and get a complete ass kicking workout in under 40 minutes. Another way would be to alternate 2 workouts over 3 non-consecutive days per week. On one day you do 500 to 1000 straight squats, on the second day you do 10 sets of alternating pull-ups and push-ups. Adjust reps and rest as needed, but keep rest short if at all. Remember this is short shock training. It has got to be hard and different then what your body is used to to get the desired result.

10 x 1 Rep

This is a technique popularized by Mike Mentzer. The idea is to do a series of 10 single max reps with the least amount of break in between the reps. This way you get a set of 10 max reps. It is basically a 10 single rep drop set. Depending on the exercise you will need 1 to 2 helpers. Also you will have to play with it a bit to set the weights ups for quick convenient strips of weight. It is much easier to use with dumbbells or weight stack machines. If you are using a weight stack machine use 2 pins. Put one at the desired weight and one just above it. This way your partner can pull the first pin and put it above the second without you stopping. You just leapfrog the pins upward. Done right 1 set is all that you will need. You might even do 2 straight sets then finish with 1 10 x 1 set.

Example:
Let us use the bench press. Since the bench is a bar exercise you will need 3 helpers. One will stand on either side of the bar and the other will spot you. If you can do this in a power rack then you will not need the spotter. Let us say your 1 rep max in the bench is 225. You will put a 45 on either side of the bar then put 4 10's and one 5 on each side of the bar. You do a rep. Hold the bar at the top. Your helpers take off a 5 from each side you do another rep. They take off a 10 and put the five back on. You work your way in this fashion down to 135. This will give you 10 single max reps. Let me emphasize if you are doing this on a regular bench you must have a spotter plus the 2 helpers for safety.

Bodyweight application:
The body weight application would be to use the hardest bodyweight exercises and/or add resistance to the body.

10 x 3

This is done just like 10 x1 except you do 3 reps with each set. You will need bigger weight drops and one set is enough. Of course you can do this with any rep range you want. Adjust the weight as necessary.

Bodyweight application:
Same as above.

6 x 6 x 6 Program

The 6 x 6 x 6 routine is six basic compound movement each performed for 6 sets of 6 reps with 2 to 3 minutes of rest between sets. It is recomended that you work into this slowly. Start with 3 non-cosequtive days and 3 sets to 6 reps. Add a set when you are able to get 6 reps in all your work sets. Once you are able to get 6 reps for all 6 sets add weight and repeat. For a natural trainee this is probably too much you may need to drop to 2 workouts per week or even 3 in 2 weeks. Or split the workout in half and alternate the routines. I will show you and exaple of each.

Example:
Let us say our 6 exercises are: barbell squat, low pully row, bench press, stiff leg dead lift, standing shoulder press, and barbell curl. Then done on one day the workout would look like:
Barbell Squat
Stiff leg Dead Lift
Barbell Row
Bench Press
Barbell Curl
Standing Shoulder Press

If you were to split this:

Workout A	Workout B
Squat	Stiff leg Dead Lift
Row	Bench Press
Curl	Shoulder Press

Bodyweight application:
1) Chose harder exercises
2) Add ressitance to the body
3) Use higher rep sets

5x5x5 Program

This is the same as the 6x6x6 Program except you pick 5 exercises and work for 5 sets of 5 reps per exercise. The progresson and split recomendations are the same.

Ultra Set

The Ultra Set is a combination of two exercises into one. Some examples are: Curl/Press, Standing Tricep extentions/press, Barbell Pullover/BenchPress, Clean or curl or reverse curl/Squat. Stifflegg Dead Lift/Regular Dead Lift, Stiff legg Dead Lift/Barbell Row.

Bodyweight applications:
Squat thrust, Burpee, Squat thrust w/ push-up, 8-count Body Builder, any of the previously mentioned exercises paired w/ pull-up, Squat/pull-up, Tiger Bend push-up/push-up, pull-up/push-up.

The Monster Maker Workout

This workout has the body builder doing a 12 to 20 rep set of clean and presses between every two exercises of their regular routine. This pattern is fallowed with all routines except arms and delts.

Bodyweight application:
Put a set of Squat Thrust, or 8-count body builders, or burpees between every two sets of exercises.

Example:

Squat, pull-up, squat thrust, push-up, sit-up, squat thrust.

One Body Part Per Workout

This is pretty straight forward. You focus on just one body part or area in a workout. Many bodybuilders follow a split that is similar to this regularily. Be careful with this because you can over train easily on this split. Since you are training a small segment of you body the tendency is to use a lot more exercises and intensity techniques which is fine for one area, but most will do this for every area because they are thinking that body part is only getting trained once per week. Which is true, but your support system is getting hit every workout. This program can be very productive, but you must listen to your body and not get carried away. Remember intesity and duration have an inverse relationship. That means as the intensity of the workout increases the duration of the workout should decrease, and rest between workouts should increase. A variation that might be better is to stay with a 3 day a week routine, and alternate between the area you are focusing on in one workout and a lower intensity workout for everything else. I also would recomend you spend some time slowly building up the intensity on your targeted area then going all out for 2 to 4 weeks. You have to be the judge here. The area being focused on can get over trained very quickly. Remember the idea is to trigger new growth. Once that happens more will only shut down growth.

Example:
Let us use a push-up specialization to illustrate how one might do this. Sart with 1 set of diamond, regular, and wide push-ups with 1 minute rest between. Now over the course of a few weeks slowly add sets until you are doing 3 sets of each type. Keep to 1 minute rest between sets. Now do 1 set of each type of push-up with 1 minute rest between them. Then finish with a giant set where you do diamond, regular, and wide for max reps of each with out a break. Spend a few workouts adapting to this then drop the single sets and go to two sets of the giant set with 1 minute rest between. Adapt to this then drop one giant set, and on your single giant set do the diamond push-ups in 21 style, do the regular push-ups in 11/2 style, and the wide with burns. The lession here is not to just copy the workout, but see how as intesity increased volume dropped.

Partial Range of Motion

This is a very powerful technique, and is how most of the great strength men of the pre steriod era built their super human strength. As a matter of fact the power rack was invented for this type of training. The basic idea is to take a weight that is much heavier then you can handle in a full range movement and move it just a small distance. Even just an inch. Or just hold it. Then over time you slowly increase the distance you move the weight.

Example:
I used Partials to develop my one arm push-up, one arm-one leg push-up, and body press. I got a 1 inch thinck board and cut it into 10 6"x6" pieces. Then I stacked the 6"x6" pieces on top of eachother. Then I would put the stack of board under my chest for the push-ups and between my hands under my head for the body press. I would lower myself the short distance to the stack of boards and push back up. Once I achieve my rep set goal. I would remove a board thus increasing the range I was traveling by 1" and build up again. Over time my range increased until I could do full range exercises.

Rep Speed

Doing reps purposely faster or slower can be a great intensity generating tool. Let's say you have been stuck on 8 reps of some exercise at a standard controled rep speed. Now you speed the cadance of the reps up and use a bit of momentum. This allows you to get 10 or even 12 with that same weight. Over time you work to slow your reps down, but at the higher rep count. A word of caution. The faster the reps the greater the momentum, and the greater the chance of injury. Does that mean not to do it? It depens. How old are you? What are your goals? Assess risk to benefit. If you are a young high school/college or elite level athlete in your prime you have do some training like this. This is how quickness and explosivness is built. But understand you will pay a price for this type of training in later years. Now if you are a 40 or 50 plus year old guy like me with beat up joints it's not a good choice.

The other side of this coin is slow rep speed. Let's use the same weight and reps as in the example above, but this time slow the reps way down. Painfully slow, Some have even strived to make one rep last a minute. Either way you are moving very slow. Take all momentum out of the exercise. Just a millimeter at a time. No matter how much your muscles burn or tremor. As a matter of fact you make the comitment to yourself that the stronger your erge is to speed up the slower you will go. At some points even stopping and holding the weight for 3 to 10 seconds to show your muscles your will is in control. After a few weeks of this you go back to the regular rep spped and that 8 rep weigh will be like nothing. You'll easily get 10 to 12 reps. This is a very safe way to train. Especially for old fart like myself, and contrary to somes belief it will not make you slower.

Example:
There are camps that recommend specific rep speeds. I find trying to move at a specific rep cadance distracts me from focusing on the muscle and decreases the intensity. So I suggest just do your reps really slow. Even stoping and holding a positon for a time. I try to really focus on the muscle and contract it one fiber at a time.

The One Minute Rep

This is an extreme version of the slow rep speed technique. This is a tactic made popular by Aurthor Jones inventor of Nautilis exercise equipment, and still championed by his protigea Elliot Darden. Basically you make one rep last one minute or longer. That one rep is one set.

Mixing Speeds

Mixing speeds is just that. Mix speeds from set to set or even with in a set.

Isometric holdes

With this you hold a positon, weight or push against an imovable object for a period of time. You can incorperate holds with other tactics or do them a lone.

Example:
The classic body weight example of this is the wall sit. You put your back against a wall, feet out in front such that your ankles are under your knees, knees are at a 90 degree angle, and the tops of your thighs are parelle to the floor. Now hold.

Negative Only Reps

This tactic is based on the priciple that people are stronger in the negative portion of an exercise. So one would load the bar with more weight then they can handle in the positive portion of an exercise and slowly do the negative portion. Generally weight trainers would need two strong spotters to do the positive portion of the exercise, but there are some tactics that a weight trainer can use by themselves. One is to use both hands to get a heavy dumbbell in place then just one to lower it. Examples of this would be using both hands to push press a dumbbell overhead then lower it with just one. Or curl dumbbell up with two hands and lower with one. For weight trainers this is a hard tactic to implement due to needing 2 to 3 spotters, but with body weight it is much easier.

Example:
With pull-ups either jump up to a chin over the bar position or use something to step up on. Once your chin is over the bar lock in and hold as long as possible. Even keep pulling as you slowly fatigue a desend. This same tactic can be used with dips. Jump or step to the straight arm position and lower slowly. With push-ups you can get in the up positon then slowly lower. Once down get on hands and knees re-set and go again. Pull-up with 2 hands and lower wtih one. Push-up with 2 hands and lower with 1. With squats lower with 1 leg and push-up with 2 or use your upper body to pull-up.

Running the Rack

Running the rack refers to a rack or sequence of dumbbells or fixed weight barbbells. There are many different ways to do this. The most common is to start at the light end and do a specific number of reps. Then, without rest, grab the next heaviest and repeat. Continue working your way up the rack in this fashion until you can't get the specific number of reps. Then work your way back down doing as many reps as you can with each weight. This is a great way to train. You have a built in warm-up. It is very intense, and efficiante. You can totally smoke a muscle or body area in just minutes.

Body weight example:
Basically you start with a light for you variaton of an exercise work your way up with harder versions, then back down.

Modified push-up, Regular push up, Feet elevated push-up, Dip, Body press, Dip, Feet elevated push-up, regular push-up, Modified push-up.

Pyramid

The Pyramid routine is used primarily with body weight exercises, but it can be used with weights. With the pyramid routine you start with a set weight, do one rep, then two reps with the same weight, and three, and on up until you can't do one more then the set before. At that point you come back down. Now you can do this with one exercise and have a break between sets, do it with a patner handing the weight back and fourth, resting only as long as it takes your partner to do his set, or by mixing one or more exercises in. The other exercises can be worked in a pyramid fashion or held at a set rep.

Bodyweight Example:
This routine was made popular by the Navy Seals. They would do pull-up, push-up, sit-up pyramids. Or pull-up, dip, sit-up, push-up pyramids. One of my favorite is pull-up, squat, push-up (or dip). This is a very challenging, result producing, and versatile routine. Well worth using.

Pull-up x 1, 2, 3, 4, 5, 6, 7, 8, 9, 10, 9, 8, 7, 6, 5, 4, 3, 2, 1
Squat   x 5, 10, 15, 20, 25, 30, 35, 40, 45, 50, 45, 40, 35, 30, 25, 20, 15, 10, 5
Push-up x 2, 4, 6, 8, 10, 12, 14, 16, 18, 20, 18, 16, 14, 12, 10, 8, 6, 4, 2

Ladders

Ladders are basically the up side of a pyramid. Usually weight trainers will use a set weight and do a rep, take a set short break, do two reps, and continue adding reps until they can't get one more rep then the set before. This is often done with a partner. They hand the weight back and fourth until one can't get the required reps. Like the pyramid routine this is very versatile, result producing, and versatile. It can be done with more then one exercise. Also you don't have to go up by one rep. It an be by any number you chose.

Eample:
One of the most challenging versions of this I've come across is to follow the patteren below with a 5 to 10 count between sets as you hold the push-up position. Keep going as long as you can get one more rep then the set before. If you can complete this it would be 55 total reps. Of course you can take a short break without holding the push-up position, but just 5 to 10 seconds. This can obviously be done with any exercise

Push-up x 1, 2, 3, 4, 5, 6, 7, 8, 9, 10

Wave

The wave routine is basically chaining together a series of pyramids. The difference is you don't max out you purposely keep the top rep low enough so you can reach it 3 or or more times. It is a tactic to increase volume. The Idea is to work at a lower intensity and a higher volume. So this would be a great change up from a cycle using a shorter higher intensity tactic or vice versa. Remember a big part of plateau breaking is switching to something different.

Example:
Pull-up x 1,2,3,2,1,2,3,2,1,2,3,2,1

Staggared Sets

Staggard sets is putting together low rep heavy weight sets with lighter weight higher weight sets. Any example of this with weights would be to do a heavy 5 rep set of curls then follow with a 15 to 20 rep set. You can also mix weight and bodyweight easily. Like a set of heavy barbbell squats followed by a high rep set of body weight squats. You can also go the other way. Light to heavy. That is very intense. This is kind of like a drop set but you want a bigger gap in reps. Low reps 5 to 10. High reps 25 to 100.

Bodyweight example:
Body press to regular or modified push-ups
one legged squat to two legged

The 50 rep set

The 50 rep set is doing 50 rep in one set. The idea is to just barerly get the 50 reps without a rest. If you need a rest then only 5 to 10 seconds. If you can get all 50 without a break then up the weight a bit. If you are unable to get the 50 then stay with that weight and work hard at eliminating the break. The application is the same for weight trainers and Body weight trainers. The only difference is the body weight trainers should use this on exercises that 50 reps would be a challenge to do.

The 100 Rep Set

This works the same as the 50 rep set, but the trainer is trying to get 100 reps.

Complete a Specific Number of Rep as Fast as Possible

This is similar to the 50 and 100 rep set, but you do get to take breaks. Your goal is to complete a predetermined amount of reps as fast as possible. Fast does not mean sloppy. You still use propper form but you try to limit your breaks and get all the reps done in the least amount of time. You can do this with one exercise or use many. Because you can take breaks and use multiple exercises the rep goal is usually 100 to 500, but you can use less. The important thing is that you challenge yourself.

Maximum Reps Completed in a Specific Tiime

This is very simular to completing a specific number of reps as fast as possible, but the focus is shifted. Here you try to get as many reps as possible in a prdetermined amount of time. So the time is constant and reps are variable where in the other tactic it's just the opposite.

The RKC Ladder

This is a great specializaton routine from the book 'Beyond Body Building' by the wicked Russian Pavel Tsatsouline. You start by performing the targeted exercise for 5 mini ladders of 1, 2, 3. Take very short rest between sets (5-10 seconds), and a minute or so between ladders. Now each time you do the routine add one ladder until you are doing 1, 2, 3 x 10. Then start with 1, 2, 3, 4 x 3. Add a ladder per workout until you are at 1, 2, 3, 4 x 6. Finally go to 1, 2, 3, 4, 5 x 2, and add a ladder per workout until you are up to 4 ladders. Now rest a few days and test the exercise you speciallized on. Weight trainers start with a weight that you can handle for 8 reps. For body weight trainees a 1, 2, 3 ladder might not be challenging enough depending on the exercise chosen and the level of the trainee. So adjust the ladder accordenly. You want the top number of the ladder to be a rep or two below half your max. So someone who's max pull-ups is 15 reps could start with a ladder of 2, 4, 6.

The Cometitive Ladder

Here is another great ladder specialization routine from 'Beyond Body Building' by Pavel. Try to keep moving from exercise to exercise. If you must rest keep it short. The numbers are set for a trainee who can do a max set of 10 pull-ups and 20 dive bomber push-ups. Adjust your weight or ladder numbers according to your fitness level and exercises chosen. The trainee will alternate between two ladders: the pull-up ladder of 1,2 3, and the dive bomber push-up ladder of 2, 4, 6. So the trainee will do 1 pull-up and go 2 db push-ups, then 2 pull-ups and 4 db push-ups, and finally 3 pull-ups and 6 db push-ups. At this point the trainee sarts back at 1 and repeats. The trainee continues this sequance until they are sure they can't get the level 3 set or acctually doesn't get it. At this point the trainee takes a one minute rest and stars the process again. This whole patteren is reapeated until the trainee can not get to level two.

BIO

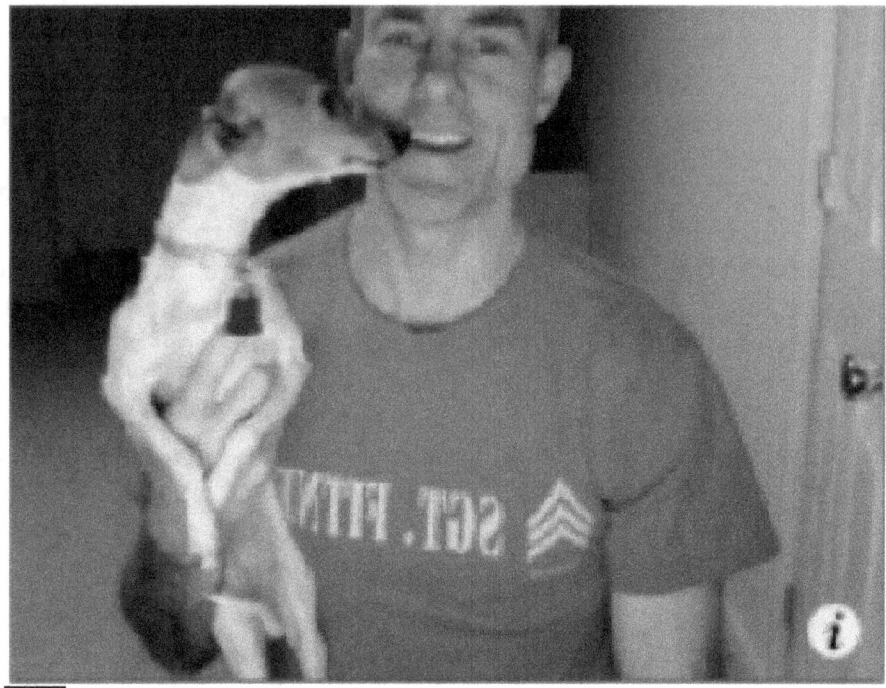

Steve Ferguson, also known as Sgt. Fitness, was born in St. Cloud, Minnesota, but is essentially a hometown boy, having lived most of his life in Fairfax County. He spent four years of service in the United States Army's elite Honor Guard (The Old Guard)., stationed at Ft. Myer, Virginia, and was called back to duty in support of Desert Storm/Shield.

Steve has 19 years of experience as a personal trainer,and is certified through the National Federation of Professional Trainers. In addition to his time in the military, his college background in psychology and independent studies has also served him well as a personal trainer. Steve credits an early fascination with the Jack LaLanne T.V. show as the catalyst for his passion with fitness.

An accomplished distance runner in his younger days, Steve came to the realization that he could be even more fit in less time, while preserving his knees, through high intensity, low impact, military-style calistentic exercises. Thus, the Sgt. Fitness style of training was born.

Steve is a career professional in vocational education at a facility that serves the needs of adults with physical and mental disAbilities in Northern Virginia. in his spare time he trains in the martial arts, likes to spend time with his dog, and is a avid fan of the cinema. A lover of the outdoors, weekends find him hiking, cycling, kayaking, and visiting nearby wineries. You can reach Sgt. Fitness at sgtfitness1@gmail.com or on youtube at sgtfitnessonline.